DEDICATION

Thank you to all the new Laser owners who asked me the questions in this booklet. It became apparent that this guide was needed, since most new owners were asking the same questions. Your questions inspired me to collate them all together for EVERYONE to benefit as well. I hope that this guide will help you navigate through the confusion and deliver a clear path to Laser success.

I would also like to shout out a huge "Thank you" and appreciation toward my life partner, who put up with hours of neglect while I pounded away on the computer. I could not do any of this without their loving support & understanding.

And of course to my pets for helping to type extra letters into this document, when they walked across the keyboard . . .

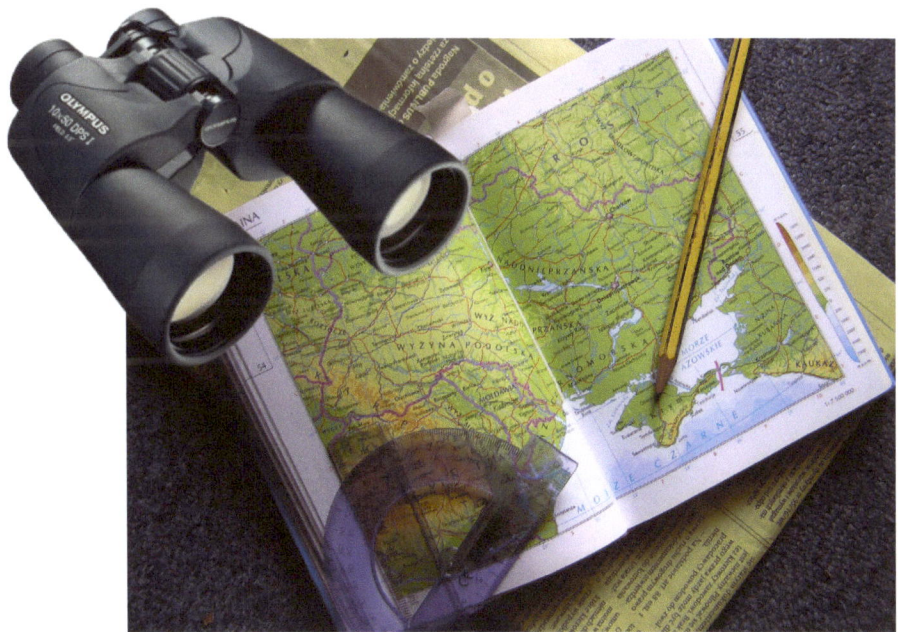

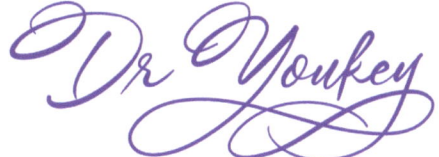

WHY READ THIS GUIDE?

Congratulations on your Laser investment! This booklet is ideal for those who are just starting out on their new Multi Radiance Medical Laser journey.

It explains how to use your Laser in simple easy-to-understand sections. You can read this manual in any order and can find the section you need in the Table of Contents.

The back section will contain some popular protocols so that you can start to use your Laser right away.

This is not meant to be a thorough discussion or explanation on Laser therapy. Instead, this is a compilation of the most Frequently Asked Questions from new Laser owners.

I hope that you find this mini guide useful - to help you navigate through the confusion and guide you toward a clear path to Laser success.

Now go help many patients live a pain-free life!

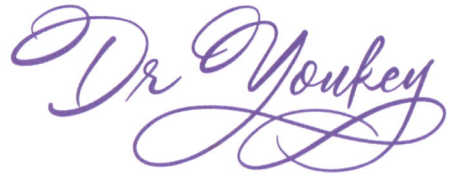

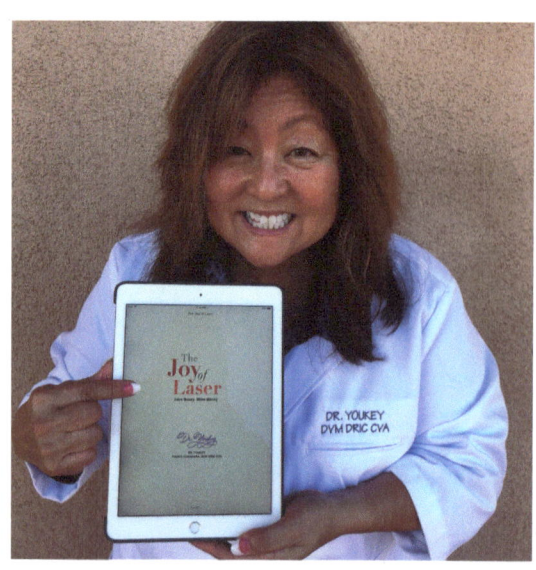

TABLE OF CONTENTS

DEDICATION	1
WHY READ THIS GUIDE?	2
DISCLAIMER	6
HOW DO I TURN MY LASER ON?	7
HOW DO I TURN ON THE BLUE LIGHT ON MY ACTIVET?	8
HOW DO I TURN OFF THE RED LIGHT?	9
IS THE RED LED JUST AN INDICATOR LIGHT?	9
I HAVE AN EMERGENCY AND HAVE TO STOP TREATMENT. HOW DO I INTERRUPT THE LASER?	10
IF I STOPPED THE TREATMENT BEFORE THE FULL TIME, WILL IT REMEMBER AND PICK UP WHERE I LEFT OFF?	10
DO I NEED TO USE THE PROBES ALL THE TIME?	11
HOW DO I CLEAN MY LASER?	12
WHAT IS THE LONGEST TIME I CAN LASER A PATIENT?	13
HOW FREQUENTLY CAN I LASER A PATIENT?	13
I FORGOT TO CHARGE THE LASER AND I HAVE TWO MORE APPOINTMENTS! WHAT CAN I DO?	14
HOW LONG DOES THE BATTERY RUN ON A SINGLE CHARGE?	14
HOW LONG DOES IT TAKE TO CHARGE THE LASER?	15
I'M NOT KEEPING TRACK OF MY LASER USEAGE. HOW DO I KNOW WHEN TO CHARGE IT?	16
WHAT IS THE LIFE OF THE LASER DIODE?	16
WHAT IS THE LOADING DOSE	17
& GENERATION RULE?	17
WHAT IS THE UNWIND PROTOCOL?	18
SHOULD I COMPRESS?	19
HOW LONG DO I USE THE PROBES ON ACUPUNCTURE POINTS?	19
HOW DO I LASER THE FACE?	20
CAN I TRAVEL WITH MY LASER?	20

WHAT ROLE DOES THE STATIC MAGNETIC FIELD PLAY?	21
WHERE DO I GET A DESICCANT TO PLACE INSIDE THE ZIPLOC® BAG?	21
HOW TIGHT DO I NEED TO SCREW IN THE PROBES?	22
I LOST ONE OF THE ACUPUNCTURE PROBES. CAN I PURCHASE THEM INDIVIDUALLY?	22
BASIC RULE SUMMARY:	23
WHICH DO I TREAT FIRST? PAIN, SWELLING OR HEALING?	24
DO I NEED TO MAKE ANY ADJUSTMENTS FOR ELDERLY OR WEAK PATIENTS?	25
WHAT IS THE 3-2-1 RULE?	26
HOW DO I LASER OVER	26
INCISION SITES?	26
WHAT ARE THE 3 REACTIONS TO LASER THERAPY TREATMENT?	27
WHAT ARE THE CONTRAINDICATIONS?	28
WHEN YOU RENT THE LASER, DO YOU ALSO RENT OUT THE PROBES?	29
HOW DO I KNOW IF MY LASER IS WORKING PROPERLY?	30
I BOUGHT TWO LASERS AND ONE HAD A FULL CHARGE WHILE THE OTHER ONE NEEDED TO BE CHARGED FOR THREE HOURS. DID I GET A USED LASER?	31
MY LASER NEEDS TO BE SHIPPED BACK FOR SERVICE. I PAID $9000 SO WILL I GET A LOANER LASER WHILE I WAIT FOR MY LASER TO BE SERVICED?	31
THE STICKER THAT COVERED A SMALL OPENING ON MY LASER CAME OFF. SHOULD I BE CONCERNED?	32
I SAW THE SAME LASER BEING SOLD ON THE INTERNET FOR A BARGAIN PRICE! WHY SHOULDN'T I PURCHASE EXTRA LASERS FROM THEM?	32
I HAVE A CLIENT WHO WANTS TO PURCHASE THE LASER. HOW DO I GO ABOUT THIS?	33
IS IT TRUE THAT I CAN RECEIVE A 10% DISCOUNT ON OVER 6000+ ACUPUNCTURE SUPPLIES?	33
SAMPLE PROTOCOLS	34
POST VACCINE & MICROCHIP PROTOCOL	34

ARTHRITIS PROTOCOL	35
HOT SPOTS (ACRAL LICK DERMATITIS) PROTOCOL	35
OTITIS PROTOCOL	36
PRE-BLOOD DRAW ANESTHETIC PROTOCOL	36
SNAKE BITES OR BITES OF UNKNOWN ORIGIN	37
POST DE-CLAW PROTOCOL	38
POST DENTAL PROTOCOL	39
ANAL SACCULITIS PROTOCOL	40
BURN PROTOCOL	41
CYSTITIS PROTOCOL	42
WANT MORE!?!	43
SURPRISE GIFT FOR YOU!	44

DISCLAIMER

Although the author and publisher have made every effort to ensure that the information in this book was correct at press time, the author and publisher do not assume and hereby disclaim any liability to any party for any loss, damage, or disruption caused by errors or omissions, whether such errors or omissions result from negligence,

This book is not intended as a substitute for the medical advice of physicians. The reader should regularly consult a physician in matters relating to his/her health and particularly with respect to any symptoms that may require diagnosis or medical attention.

The information in this book is meant to supplement, not replace, proper professional medical care. Like any medical equipment, Lasers poses some inherent risk. The authors and publisher advise readers to take full responsibility for their safety and know their equipment and precautions necessary to prevent harm to the operator or patients. Before practicing the skills described in this book, be sure that your equipment is well maintained, and do not take risks beyond your level of experience, aptitude, training, and comfort level.

Protocols and suggestions presented in this book is solely from the Author. No Laser company endorses the protocols or how to use the Laser presented in this book. The protocols are presented for entertainment purposes only and not meant to diagnose or treat any conditions.

Laser therapy should not be commenced until a diagnosis is reached and used only under the direct or indirect supervision of your physician.

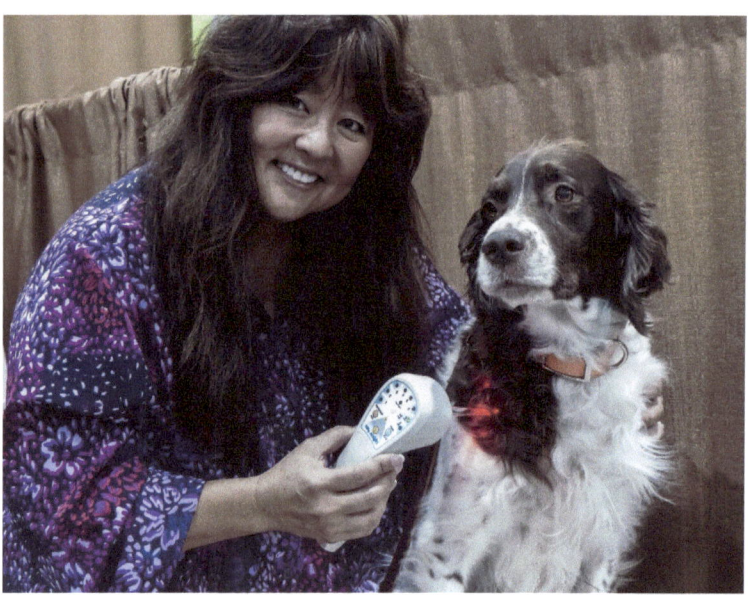

Copyright © 2020 DR YOUKEY LASERRIFFIC

The contents of this book is copyrighted and all rights are reserved. No part of this book may be reproduced or transmitted in any form or by any means, electronic or mechanical, including photocopying, recording, or by any information storage and retrieval system, without written permission in writing from the author.

HOW DO I TURN MY LASER ON?

It's always good to get in the habit of covering the opening of the Laser with the palm of your hand before starting it up. You need to occlude all light while it goes through it's self-test when the Laser is cold.

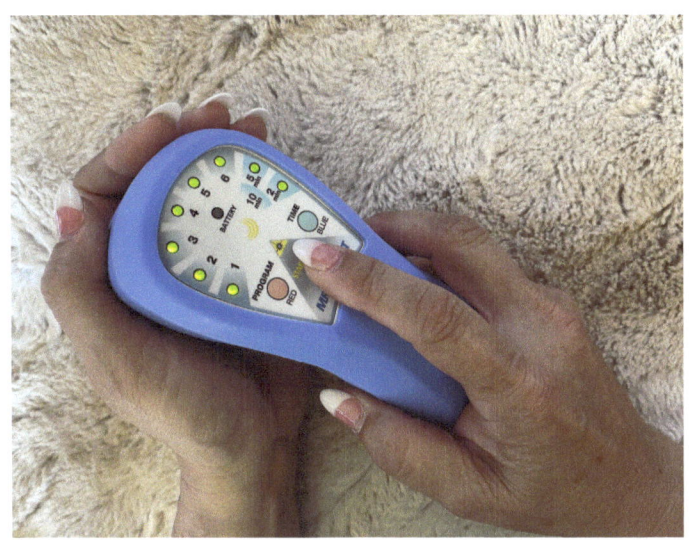

Start by placing the opening in your palm. With your other hand, long press the on/off or start/stop button until all the lights come on. Then let go that button. You will see that all the lights are on. Now it is ready to run the self-test and calibration. Keeping the opening occluded from light, now short press the same button. You will see that the Laser is now going through its self diagnostic. If the Laser is already warmed up, it will not need to go through this step again. After it finishes the self diagnostic, it will default on 50 Hz (program 1) on the Activet and 5 Hz on the TQ Solo. Your Laser is now ready to use.

Some newer models of Pain Away or My Pet Laser has shortened this second step. Simply press the on/off button for two seconds while covering the opening and the Laser will undergo its self-test.

For the PRO or Shower, follow the directions on the screen while covering the opening. It is not necessary to do a self-test each time you use the Laser.

HOW DO I TURN ON THE BLUE LIGHT ON MY ACTIVET?

While the Laser is running a program and "on" (flashing red), you can simply press the blue (timer) button. By depressing this button while the unit is running, you can turn the blue light off and on. You cannot turn the blue light on if the Laser is not running a program.

You can choose to have the blue light on or off at will. This picture shows a tiger receiving blue light treatment to help reduce bacterial load and MRSA prior to releasing back into its' enclosure.

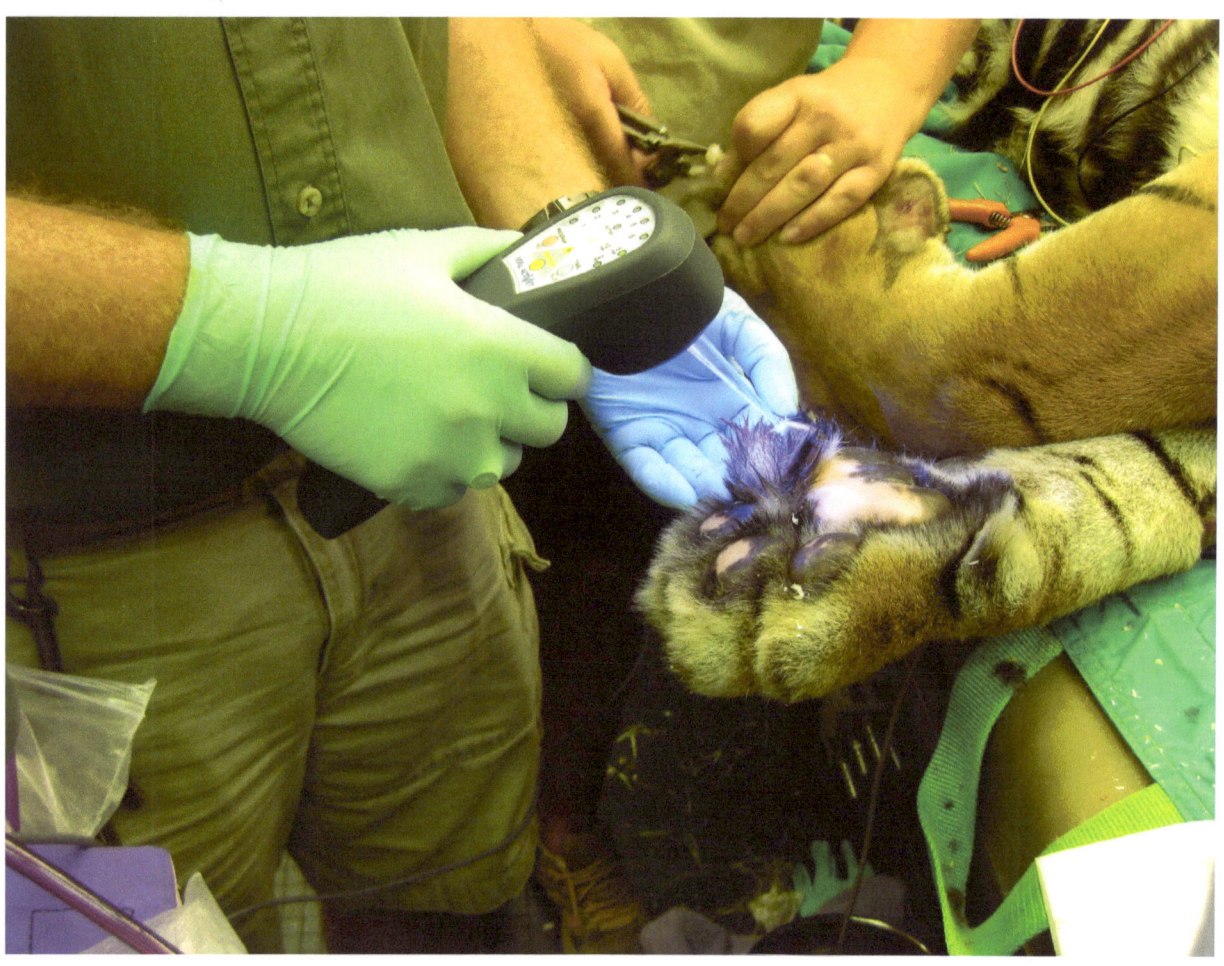

HOW DO I TURN OFF THE RED LIGHT?

On the Activet, for many instances (like when Lasering a cat) I like to turn off the red LED light. This is especially true when Lasering the facial points if using the acupuncture probes. While the Laser in running and flashing red, simply press the red button and you can turn the red LED off and on. You cannot turn off the red LED on the TQ Solo, Pain Away or My Pet Laser.

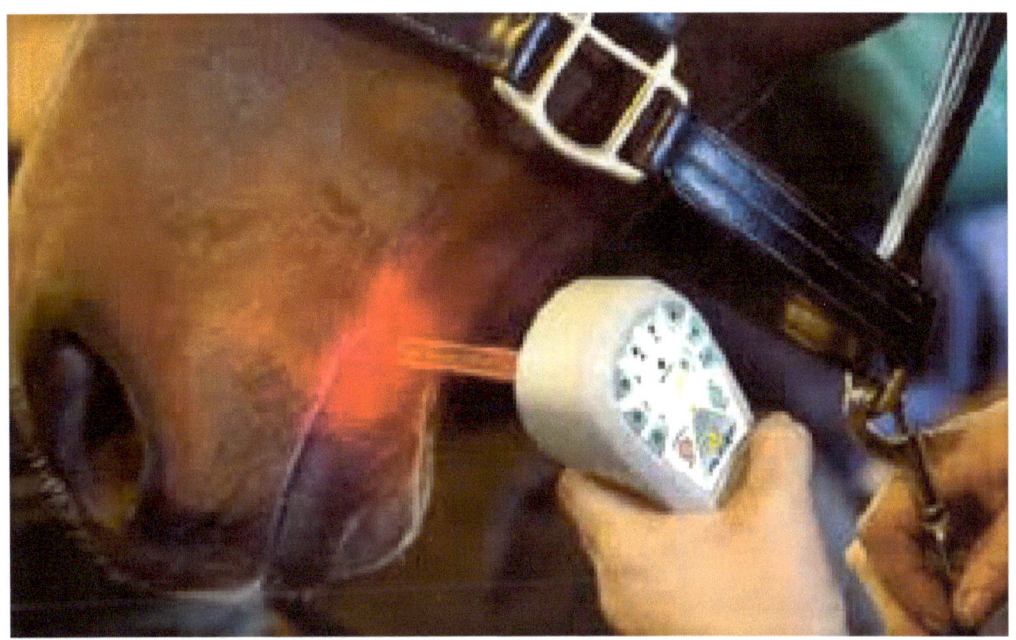

IS THE RED LED JUST AN INDICATOR LIGHT?

No. The red LED at 640 nm does help to reduce inflammation as well as to act as an indicator light to let you know that the Laser is on. Also, after using the Laser for awhile, the red LED will give off a soothing gentle warmth which feels good for arthritic patients.

I HAVE AN EMERGENCY AND HAVE TO STOP TREATMENT. HOW DO I INTERRUPT THE LASER?

Simply push the on/off start/stop button. This will stop the Laser treatment.

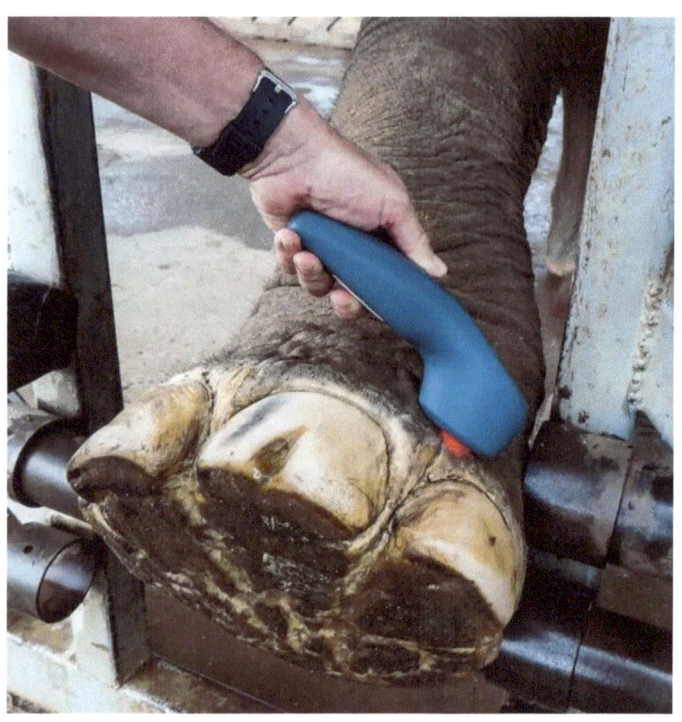

IF I STOPPED THE TREATMENT BEFORE THE FULL TIME, WILL IT REMEMBER AND PICK UP WHERE I LEFT OFF?

No. It will reset and start again. The Laser does not have a memory of it's count-down once you interrupt the program cycle.

DO I NEED TO USE THE PROBES ALL THE TIME?

No. I only use the probes for certain situations or when I am doing Laser-Acupuncture. I use the wound probe to make it easier to glide over my own face when doing facials and anti-aging procedures. I also use the wound probe to protect the Laser occasionally from a dirty environment. But I would rather put the Laser inside a disposable Ziploc® baggie if the area I am Lasering is dirty of infectious.

For arthritis, do not cover the opening with the wound probe. The probes will prevent the gentle warmth from reaching the muscles to help aid in pain relief.

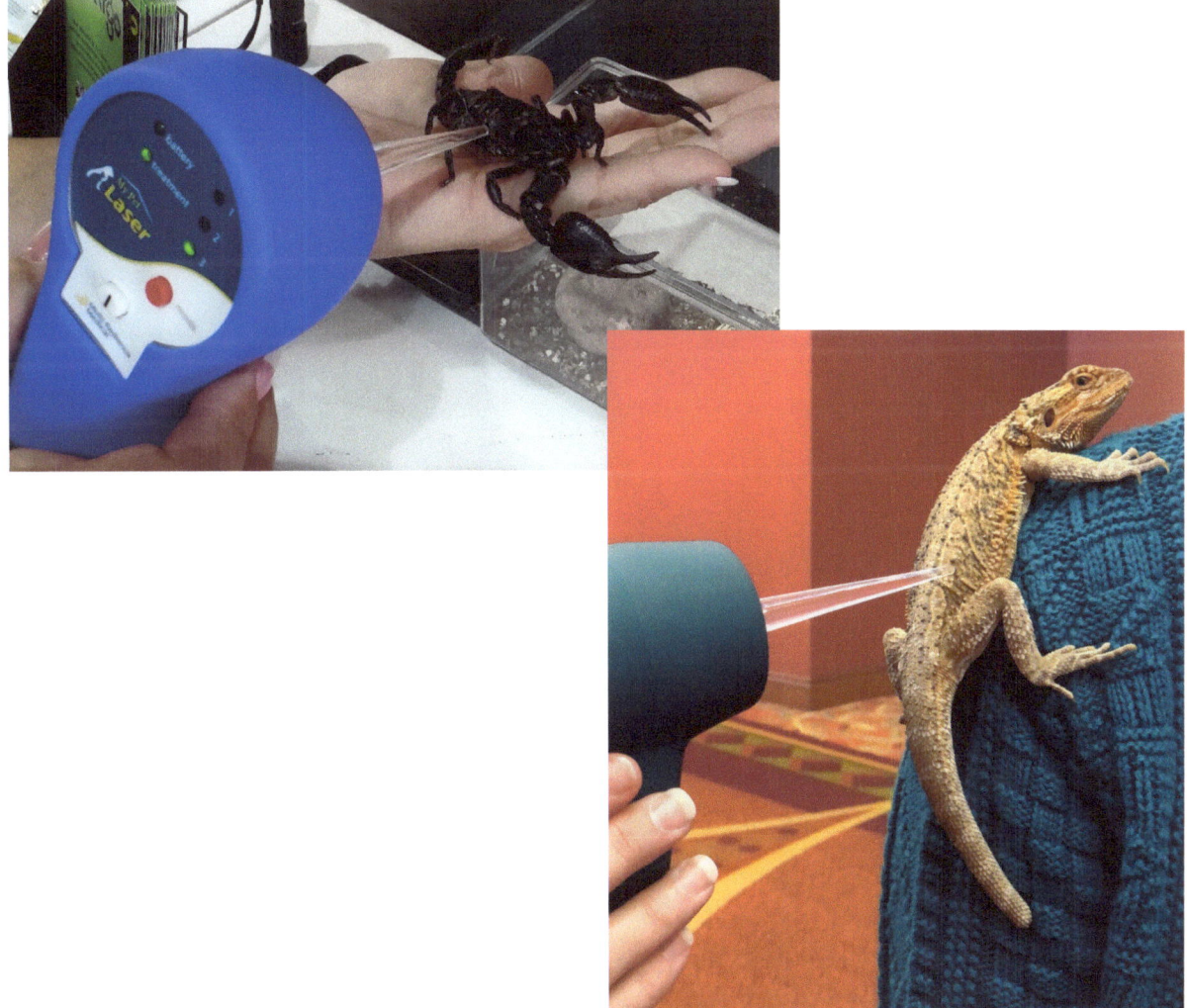

HOW DO I CLEAN MY LASER?

Your Laser is an investment and I would not use products that could degrade the plastic with anything containing alcohol. Alcohol can also dry out the probes and cause them to crack. It can also age plastic faster than normal.

I recommend a wipe called Certol. This is a plastic sterilizer that not only cleans but also kills bacteria and even pseudomonas. You can purchase Certol wipes from your veterinary supply distributor or on Amazon.

In a pinch, you can also use any screen wipe that does not contain alcohol or other chemicals known to be harmful to plastic.

Make sure that you remove the silicone cover occasionally and wipe down the Laser. You also want to be sure that the lens remain clear and not cloudy.

You can order replacement silicone covers if you ever need to. They now come in a selection of colors depending on the model of your Laser.

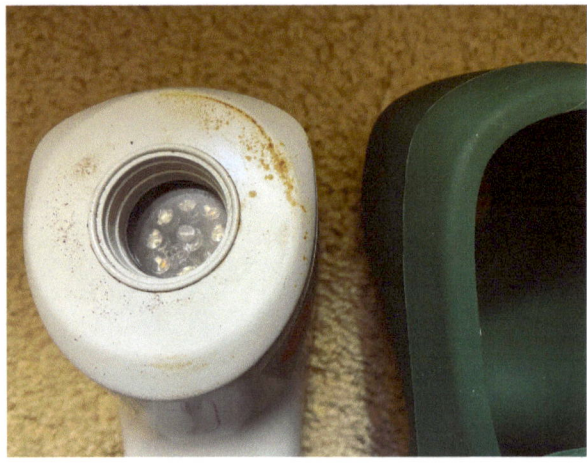
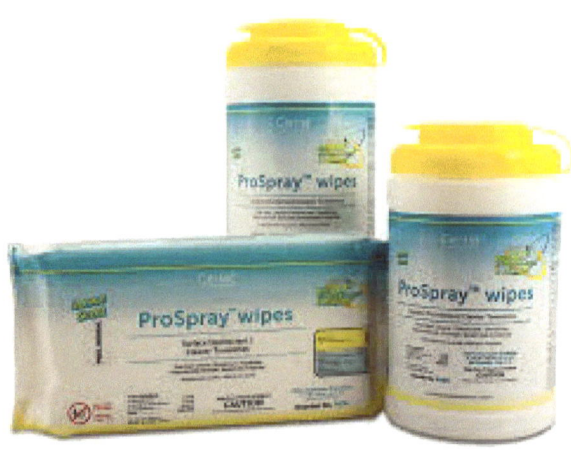

WHAT IS THE LONGEST TIME I CAN LASER A PATIENT?

You can Laser up to 40 minutes total body in a single session if there are multiple areas that need to be addressed i.e. ear infection, hip problems, hot spot. Less time for elderly or delicate / weak / fragile patients. You should limit the total time on the face to 10 minutes. And limit to 5 minutes over the thyroids.

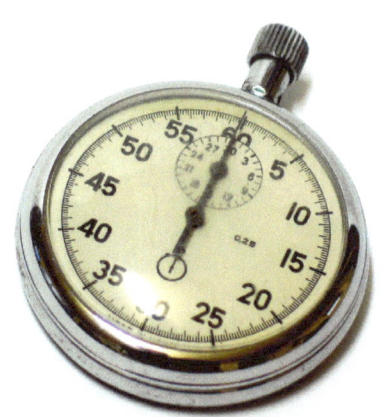

The reason why you don't go over 40 minutes is that the body needs to rest after being Lasered for that long. You aren't doing any harm - but you aren't giving any benefit either. You are simply wasting your Laser diodes life as well as your time.

And remember that rule of 5 minutes to reduce pain and 2 minutes to heal. Lasering more than that doesn't mean you will get better results.

HOW FREQUENTLY CAN I LASER A PATIENT?

You can Laser every 4 hours in severe cases such as burns, snake bites and chronic situations. If the patient starts to experience pain, we need to back off and not Laser that often,

Every patient reacts differently and some will react faster to Laser light therapy. This is where your medical expertise will come into play as adjustments will need to be made.

I FORGOT TO CHARGE THE LASER AND I HAVE TWO MORE APPOINTMENTS! WHAT CAN I DO?

Luckily, some the Laser models can run with the charger cord plugged in! So in an emergency situation where you think the Laser will run out of battery life during a treatment, simply plug it into the wall and you can continue to Laser. Now instead of being cordless, you now have a corded device.

This works on the Pain Away, My Pet Laser, Activet and Activ models.

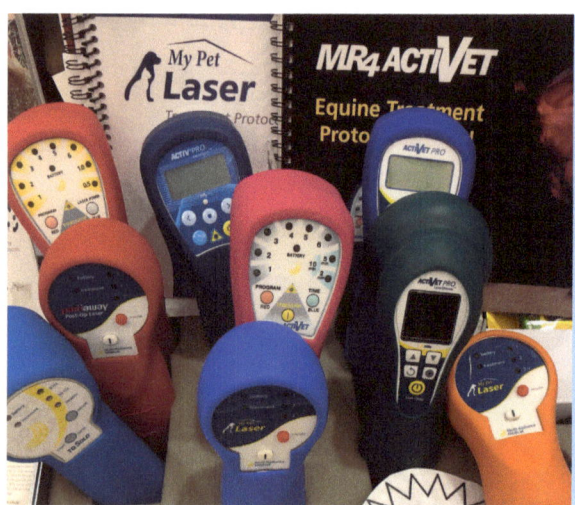

HOW LONG DOES THE BATTERY RUN ON A SINGLE CHARGE?

This depends on the Laser model and how it was used. Some programs take more energy than others. Were both the red and blue LED lights used?

In general, you can expect about 7 hours "on" for the Shower & PRO models, 8 hours "on" for the Activet & Activ models, and 18 hours for the TQ Solo, My Pet Laser and the Pain away!

HOW LONG DOES IT TAKE TO CHARGE THE LASER?

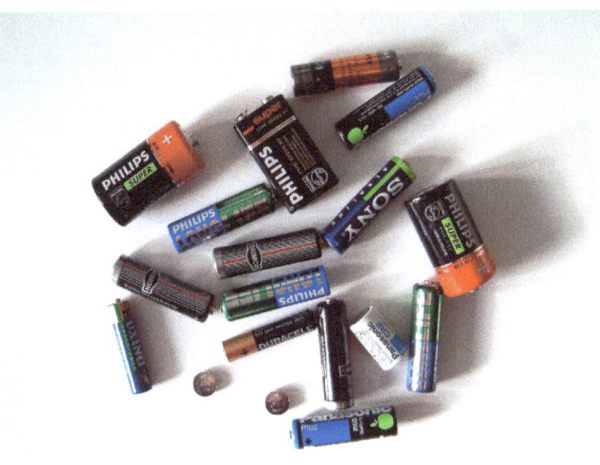

It depends on the how discharged it is. When you plug the charger in, the battery indicator light will be red. As soon as the Laser is charged full, this light will turn green. It is now time to remove the charger from the wall and Laser.

If the Laser is completely discharged, it may take up to 3 hours to charge back to full.

It's best to let the battery run down a bit. Do not keep it plugged into the charger and the wall all the time. This will shorten the life of the battery.

The batteries are constantly on a slow trickle down charge. So if you haven't used the Laser in a while, it will once again be red when you plug the charger back in.

The battery cannot be replaced on your own. If your battery ever needs to be replaced, simply contact me for instructions and approximate cost. My own Lasers are going on 9+ years without the need for replacement batteries!

I'M NOT KEEPING TRACK OF MY LASER USEAGE. HOW DO I KNOW WHEN TO CHARGE IT?

The Activet, Activ, My Pet Laser and Pain Away Lasers will begin to turn itself off after finishing a treatment or the battery light will begin to flash red once when the treatment session is finished. Sometimes it won't signal the end of the treatment with a beep. And with other models, you will see a flash of red when you first turn on the Laser. You don't need to wait until the Laser is completely discharged to begin charging. Just unplug it once the Laser is fully charged.

For the PRO & Shower Models, there is a convenient built-in battery meter on the screen so you know exactly how much life is left.

WHAT IS THE LIFE OF THE LASER DIODE?

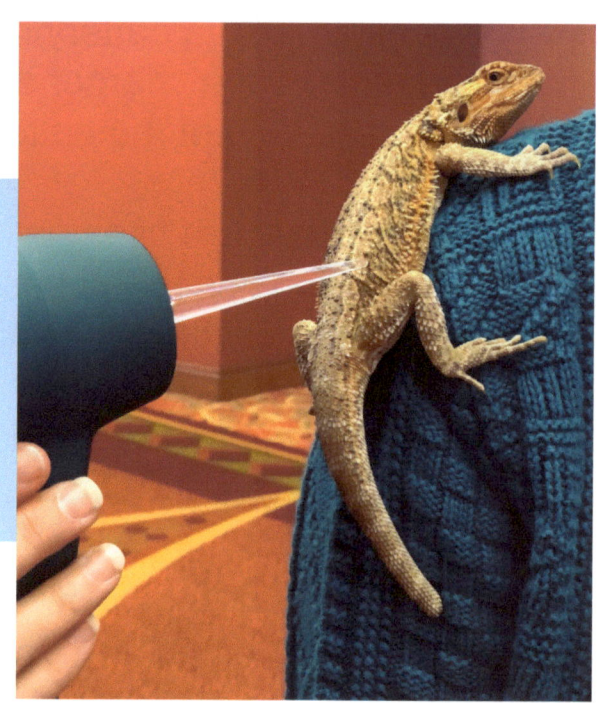

10,000 hours "on". Or 416.66666 days "on" 24/7! That's a long time.

WHAT IS THE LOADING DOSE & GENERATION RULE?

Many people want to know when they will start to see benefits. This happens when you reach the LOADING DOSE. This is the amount of Laser treatments needed to see an effect. Once the LOADING DOSE is reached, patients will feel 10 - 40% reduction in pain.

The LOADING DOSE is similar to how antibiotics work in the body. One pill will usually not show improvement but as the drug accumulates in the body and reaches that LOADING DOSE - the patient will begin to receive therapeutic benefit. Depending on the drug, you usually do not take just one antibiotic pill. Same with the Laser as it is additive as well. You don't just perform one Laser therapy session either.

People still want to know when this usually happens and it differs with each patient depending on the cause of the issue. But in general we can estimate the GENERATION RULE. If you are in your thirties, it may take three weeks to resolve the chronic pain. This way you can gauge how long it will take a patient to achieve full benefits. For acute pain, the faster you Laser, the sooner the pain relief.

An example of acute injury is with a twisted ankle - you want to Laser the moment it happens. If you start Laser treatments immediately, it is as if the ankle didn't twist at all.

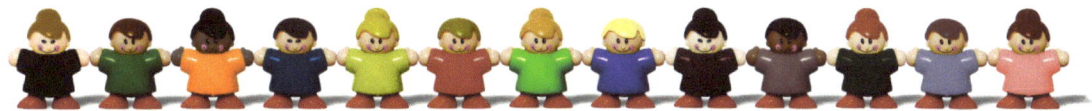

WHAT IS THE UNWIND PROTOCOL?

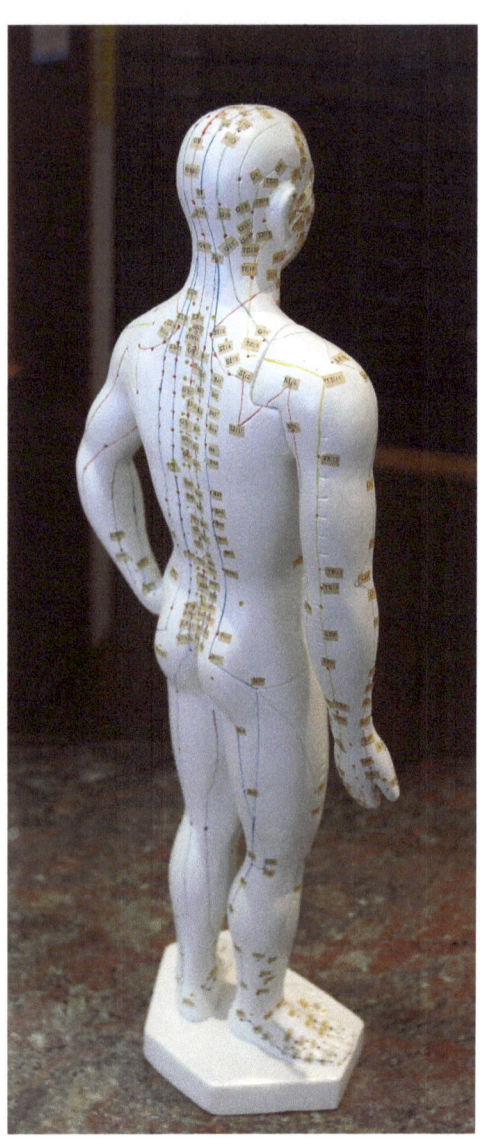

In acupuncture, there are inner and outer bladder lines on each side of the spinal column. This is where the nerve roots are appearing between the muscles (latissimus dorsi and longisimus muscles).

If you Laser for two minutes along the associated nerves affecting the area, you will have a much better treatment outcome. Then after you do this unwind protocol, go to the area that needs treatment. The unwind protocol does several things: it stops the pain cascade to the brain by activating the gate theory, releases endorphins and natural serotonins within the body.

To scan correctly, run the Laser from the base of the skull to the top of the tail head at a very slow 1 cm / sec advance with the Laser head directly on the fur. You will want to do this scan once or twice.

Use 1000 Hz if you are Lasering to reduce pain (sedate) as in arthritic cases. Most of the time, you will be using this frequency.

Use 50 Hz if you are Lasering to heal a wound (tonify).

SHOULD I COMPRESS?

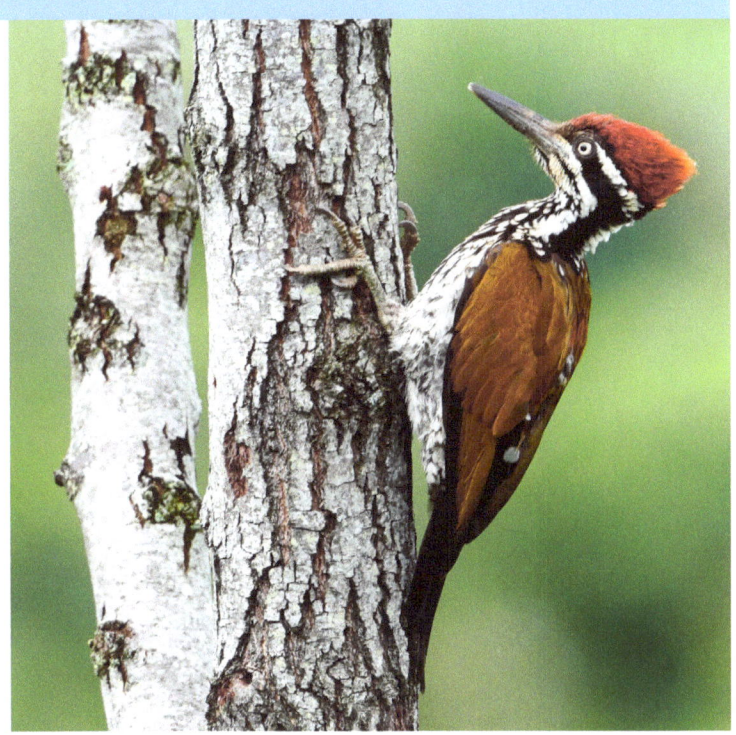

Yes, if the patient & Lasering area can tolerate it. Gentle compression (also known as the Woodpecker Method) will help to push away the blood which is a barrier. When you are able to push away the blood in heavily muscular areas, this will help to drive the Laser photons deeper into the tissues. Do not compress over wounds or with the probes.

It is not necessary to push the probes into the patient. It is the energy of the light itself that is stimulating the acupuncture points.

HOW LONG DO I USE THE PROBES ON ACUPUNCTURE POINTS?

15 - 30 seconds for smaller animals, up to 3 minutes for large animals. You can also repeat the points. You can also do a combination of traditional needles, EA and Laser at the same time. For example, you can place GV 20 in place, then work on the other points with the Laser. Laser-acupuncture is excellent for points directly over delicate structures or organs.

HOW DO I LASER THE FACE?

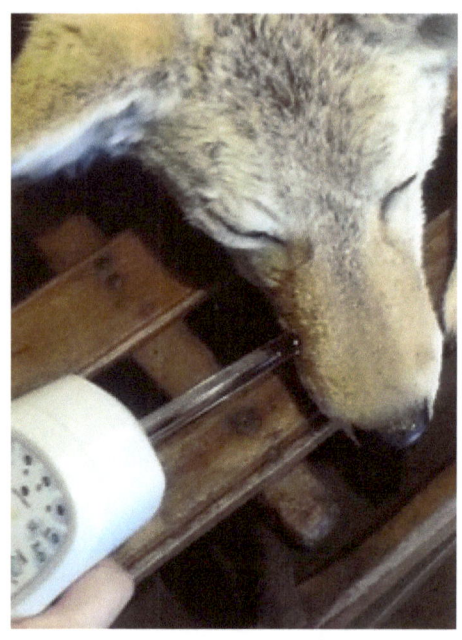

I always turn off the LED's when I am Lasering the face. The LED light is not collimated so it will radiate out in all directions, making it irritating for the patients' eyes. You do not need the LED to do the job as it is the invisible Laser photons that is important and doing most of the work (photobiomodulation). I never aim toward the eye as there will not be a blink reflex with the actual Laser 905 nm Super Pulsed Laser beam.

Unfortunately, the Pain Away, TQ Solo and My Pet Lasers do not have the ability to turn off the LED lights. So be sure that the light is not aimed directly toward the eyes or retina. You can use the included goggles to help shield the eyes if you wish.

CAN I TRAVEL WITH MY LASER?

I travel world-wide with my Lasers! Your MRM Lasers are rated Class IM safe, allowing travel anywhere around the world. The rating is on the label located on the handle (underneath the silicone cover). Be sure to carry it on, rather than checking it in with baggage. It's always safer to carry it with you. I tuck my Laser into a small carry pouch with my probe and charger.

WHAT ROLE DOES THE STATIC MAGNETIC FIELD PLAY?

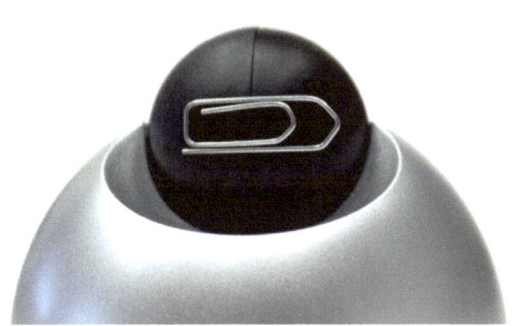

The magnetic field helps to collimate the Laser beam which is very important when using the probes and doing Laser acupuncture. The magnets also keep the nitric oxide disassociated from the cytochrome-c oxidase enzyme. The free nitric oxide helps reduce inflammation while keeping vasodilation active. The magnetic field should be kept 5 inches away from a pacemaker.

It also makes a handy paper clip picker-upper!

WHERE DO I GET A DESICCANT TO PLACE INSIDE THE ZIPLOC® BAG?

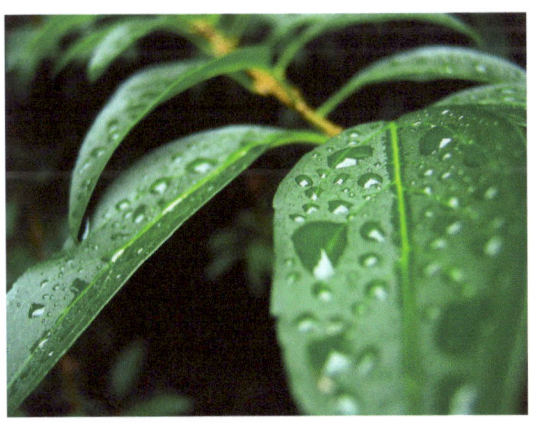

Desiccant packs placed inside the baggie will help to absorb any moisture preventing damage to the Laser when using in moist, humid or wet environments. Start saving them from prescription bottles and ask your staff to start collecting them from Oriental rice crackers and cookie bags. This is more economical when compared to the expensive desiccants sold at camera stores. You can also purchase packs at Amazon.

HOW TIGHT DO I NEED TO SCREW IN THE PROBES?

Not tight at all! Just enough to hold them in place. If you over tighten, it may become stuck or you may strip the threads. If it does get stuck, use the rubber can opener pad, duct tape or silicone lid on the wound probe to help remove them.

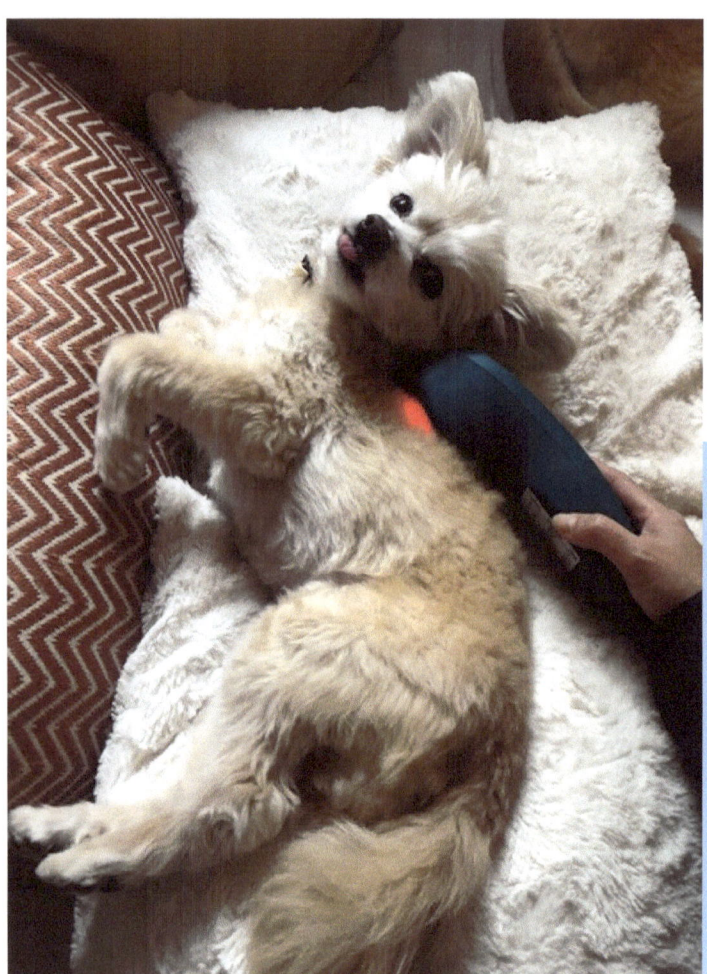

I LOST ONE OF THE ACUPUNCTURE PROBES. CAN I PURCHASE THEM INDIVIDUALLY?

Yes and no. They are sold in a set of 4 with the protective cases for $500 plus shipping. Take care of them like any other medical device accessory and do not use anything that has alcohol in it as it will crack the probe and void the warranty. The probes may also be cleaned with Certol wipes. The dome probe is available separately for $99. Sometimes there are specials on them, so please ask me.

BASIC RULE SUMMARY:

My three most used and first "go-to" programs:
Pain relief: Any frequency over 1000 Hz. I like 1000 Hz.
Pain with swelling: 1000 - 3000 Hz
Healing: 50 Hz

Any program over 1000 Hz is to control pain.
Any program below 500 Hz is to speed healing.

DO NOT mix healing and pain control on the same area at the same treatment session. This would be like trying to boil water for 2 minutes and then trying to freeze that water for 2 minutes. The net result is zero - you neither boiled nor froze the water. However, you may mix similar programs such as 1000 Hz, 1000-3000 Hz, 5000 Hz. You can mix "like" programs for resistant cases by alternating each treatment with similar frequencies.

You can also switch between pain relief and healing after 4 hours.

Older or fragile patients will require less treatment time. Patients with less mass will take less time than a patient with more mass.

You always start out with more treatments and longer treatment times initially to reach the loading dose, then taper off as you start to see progress.

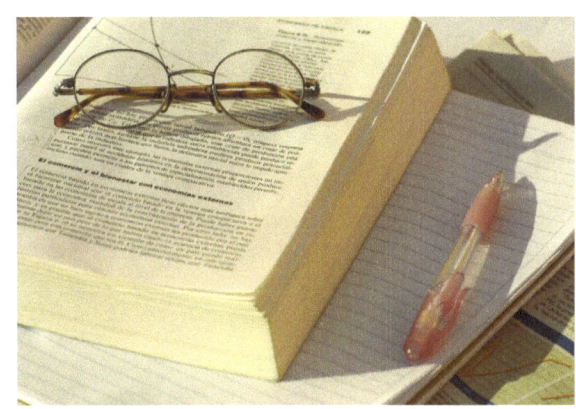

2 minutes to heal
5 minutes to stop pain

WHICH DO I TREAT FIRST? PAIN, SWELLING OR HEALING?

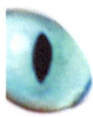 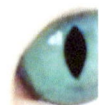

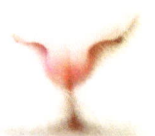

When presented with a patient that has all three things going on: pain, swelling and the need to heal, which program do you start with first?

Follow the Priority Principle when this happens. This actually occurs frequently as in a case of post op surgery. There is both pain and swelling, but also needs to heal at the tissue level.

Priority Principle says to always attack the pain & swelling first with 1000 Hz - 3000 Hz for five minutes. The reason for this choice is simple - you need to reduce the pain and swelling for the patient to heal. When the patient is in pain, it is hard for the body to heal.

Lower frequencies such as 50 Hz actually cause more circulation to surge into the area being Lasered. This can cause more pain! If the area is already in pain or swollen, this choice will cause more pain.

Yet you worry about the healing - not to worry - as ALL the frequencies are actually healing at the cellular level. You are just adjusting the depth and the circulation with the choice of frequencies. Photobiomodulation is occurring at all Hz.

When there is no more pain or swelling, you can now switch to 50 Hz to promote healing since it brings in more healing factors with the increased circulation.

If you find that this causes pain, switch back to the pain reduction mode. This is where the "Art of Medicine" will come into play and you will need to adjust your protocols.

DO I NEED TO MAKE ANY ADJUSTMENTS FOR ELDERLY OR WEAK PATIENTS?

Yes! Older or weak patients take much less time and frequency of treatments. If you normally like to Laser for five minutes, back down to two minutes. This is also true for smaller young patients as well. The less mass; the less time & frequency of treatments. These patients react to the Laser treatments quickly and it is easier to give them too much photonic energy.

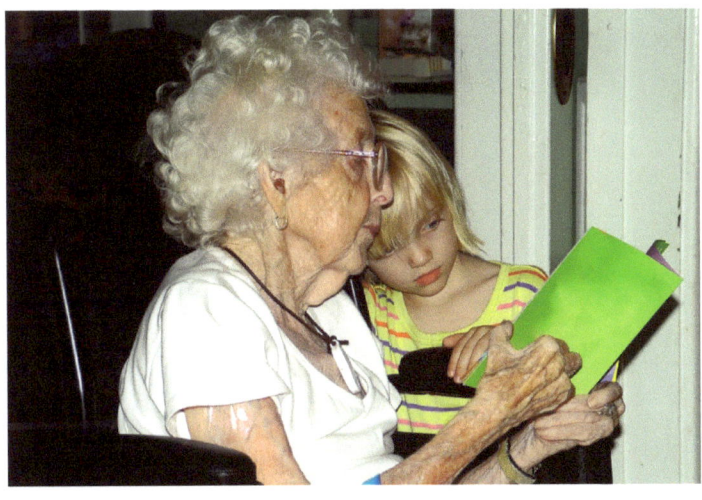

Also some disease conditions such as MS patients reacts much faster to light therapy. So reduce the time of treatment greatly. Adjust the time, depending on the response of the patient.

Be sure to avoid the GROWTH PLATES in very young patients as well. We don't want to accelerate growth in one limb!

Finally, for patients who are sensitive to flashing lights (such as epileptic patients) turn off the LED lights. We don't want to induce any unwanted seizures!

WHAT IS THE 3-2-1 RULE?

For most paying clients, I usually start with a schedule of 3 times the first week, 2 times the second week, and re-access to see if I can reduce down to 1 time the third week. Depending on how the patient responds you may need to adjust this schedule. Some patients respond faster and may not need all the sessions. Other chronic conditions will need more sessions initially to reach the loading dose.

HOW DO I LASER OVER INCISION SITES?

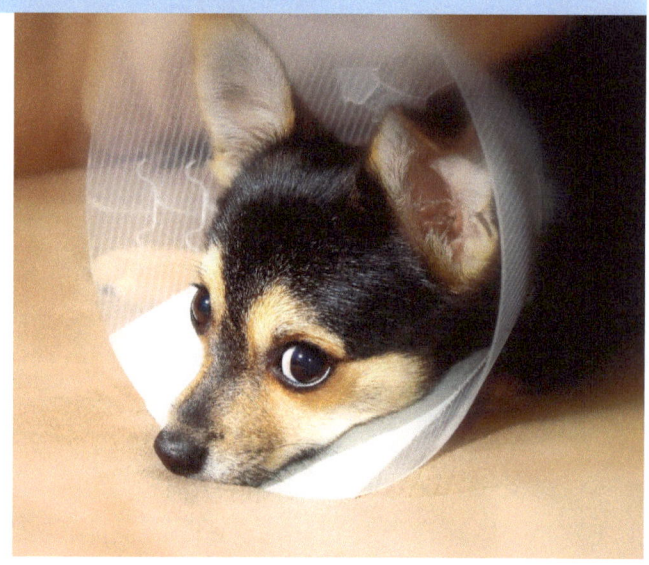

Start in the periphery and work your way slowly to the middle where the suture line is. Laser at a slow 1 cm / sec scan and as close to the surface without touching it. Use the blue light to kill any incidental bacteria that my have been introduced into the incision area. This should take less than a minute to complete.

If you need the incision to weep (such as cases where there is a drain), do not Laser directly over the incision area. It will heal too fast and the drain will not remain patent.

Do Laser over bruised areas surrounding the incision to help heal them faster.

WHAT ARE THE 3 REACTIONS TO LASER THERAPY TREATMENT?

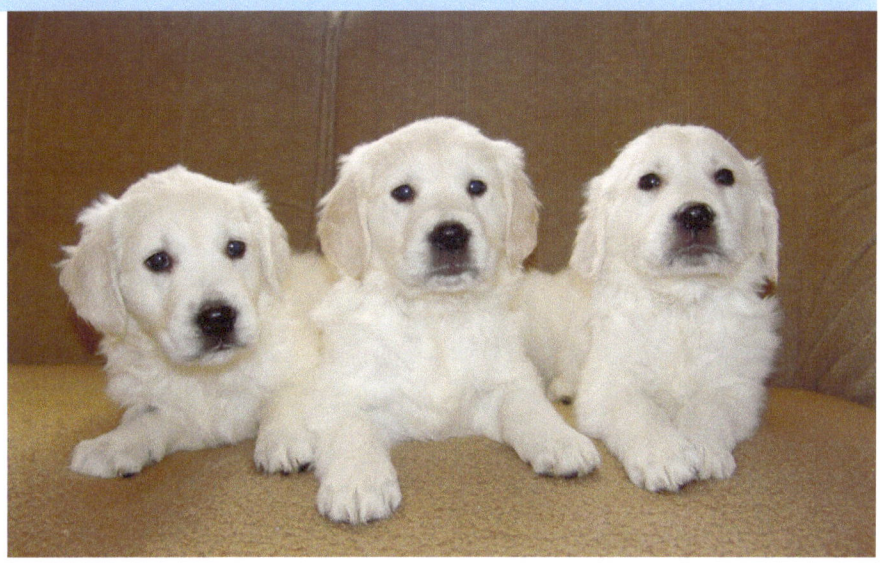

1) The first reaction is - Nothing. We haven't reached the loading dose yet. Much like antibiotics and acupuncture, it takes more sessions early on and then we can taper off as the loading dose is reached and we see improvement.

2) They may experience some pain. This is due to increased circulation in the area. This isn't a bad thing as the cells reacted positively to the Laser therapy and started to increase circulation. It is healing at the cellular level. Wait until the pain subsides and the circulation decreases before Lasering again. Some patients react faster than other. Make a note of this in the records and next time treat with less time and make sure that you are using the pain reduction program (above 1000 Hz).

3) 10 - 40% reduction in pain, each and every time you Laser! This is the reaction I would like all patients to have. When this starts to happen, you can start to reduce the time and frequency of Laser treatments. You have successfully reached the loading dose and we can now start to taper off (much like pred).

WHAT ARE THE CONTRAINDICATIONS?

1) Do not Laser directly into the eye. There is however a safety factor of 30 seconds should you inadvertently flash someone with the Laser.
2) Pregnancy - do not Laser directly over the fetus. This is not because it's dangerous, but because currently there are not enough case studies that says it is safe. So we want to err on the side of caution.
3) Do not Laser on growth plates (epiphysis). We don't want to accelerate uneven growth.
4) Stop the bleeding first. This is because we will be increasing the circulation into the area so you want to be sure that the clotting factors have already set in.
5) Epileptic patients - for people sensitive to flashing light, turn the flashing LED's off for them.
6) People who are allergic to light. This is a rare condition, however, there are some people who are allergic to being in contact with any light.
7) Medications that increase sensitivity to light therapy. Reduce the amount of treatment time if the patient is taking any medications that affect the skins sensitivity to light.
8) Cancerous masses - currently, we will err on the side of caution and not Laser over known malignant masses. However, this precaution may someday be lifted as more studies are showing positive results of Laser increasing ones own immune response to fight cancer.
9) Reduce the fever first. If the patient has a fever - this indicates that there is an ongoing infection within the body. Because Laser therapy increases circulation, we don't want to spread the infection or possibly contribute to a systemic infection so please give appropriate antibiotics and wait a few days prior to initiating Laser treatment.
10) Steroid injection - because the steroids will mask the effect of Laser therapy, wait 72 hours to begin Laser treatment. It won't hurt to Laser, you just won't see any benefit.

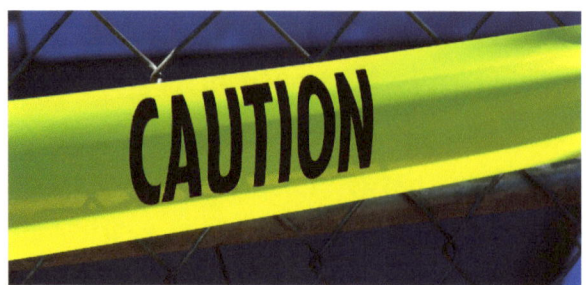

WHEN YOU RENT THE LASER, DO YOU ALSO RENT OUT THE PROBES?

No. I do not rent out the probes. I do not want untrained people to do Laser acupuncture. I just want them to "paint" and I instruct them thoroughly on how to use it correctly. There are acupuncture points that I do not want stimulated that can cause adverse reactions in the patient. Plus, I cannot purchase the probes separately so I don't want to lose them either!

I rent my Laser out to my good existing clients. I also get a deposit for the entire retail MSRP amount should they either damage the Laser or wish to purchase it after the rental period. The rental agreement in Excel format is in your dropbox. You just need to input your own practice information.

If the rental is less than a week, do not send home the charger. The replacement charger is also quite expensive, although you can deduct that amount from your deposit.

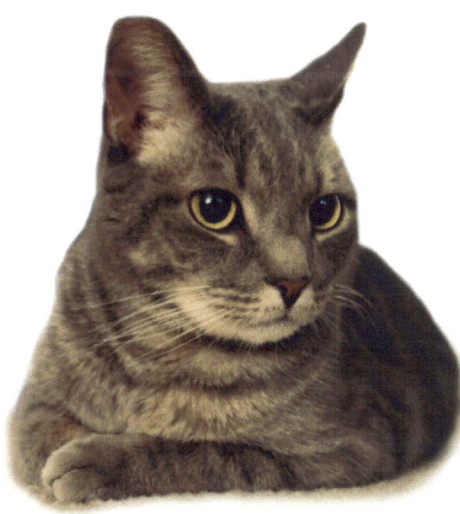

Other hospitals have a unique method of renting the Laser in-house. The clients are shown how to use the Laser and they purchase a reduced rental bundle. They make a rental appointment and come into the hospital to use the Laser. There is no tech time and the clients save money by Lasering their pet themselves. Be sure that your clients sign a consent and liability waiver.

HOW DO I KNOW IF MY LASER IS WORKING PROPERLY?

If the Laser passes the self-diagnostic check when you first turn it on, it is working. If your Laser is not passing the self-diagnostic then it is time to have your Laser checked.

Your Laser should also make a slight distinct sound on each program. If you don't hear any sound on any program, I would have the Laser diagnosed. You can apply a stethoscope against the Laser if you have a hard time hearing the different sounds.

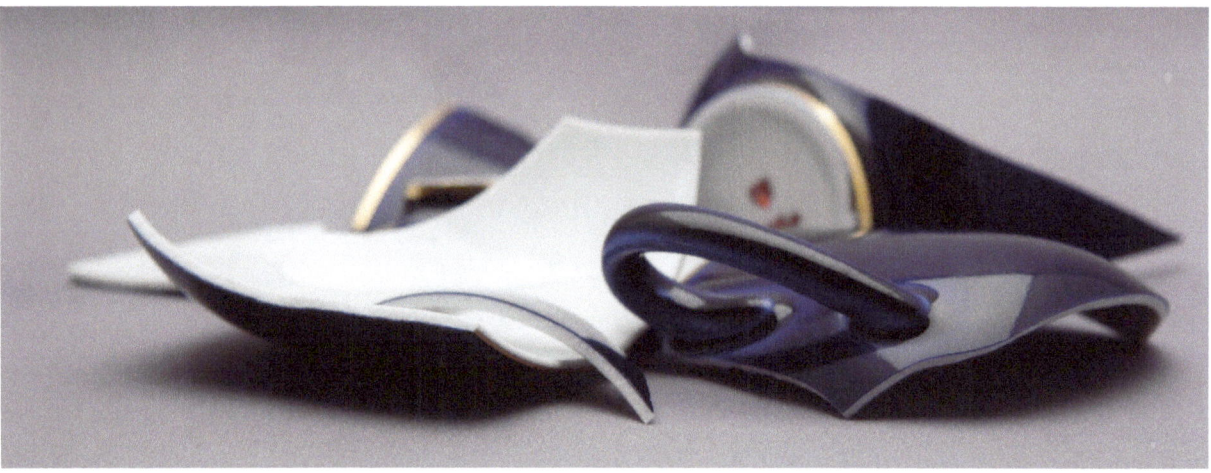

If you need service on your Laser, contact me so that I can request an RMA (Return Merchandise Authorization) from the company. Any equipment being shipped back needs this number so that the service department knows what to do with your Laser. Do not ship it back without this number both in the box as well as prominently labeled on the outside of the box.

Sometimes, the service department can trouble shoot over the phone and may be able to help you without having to ship the Laser back to Ohio. Either way, please contact me so that I can coordinate and help you.

I BOUGHT TWO LASERS AND ONE HAD A FULL CHARGE WHILE THE OTHER ONE NEEDED TO BE CHARGED FOR THREE HOURS. DID I GET A USED LASER?

No. We don't sell used or refurbished Lasers as new. All Lasers are shipped new from Ohio direct from the manufacturer; however, each Laser may have a different amount of charge in them. This is due to the assembly line fashion of the Lasers before it is calibrated and shipped out.

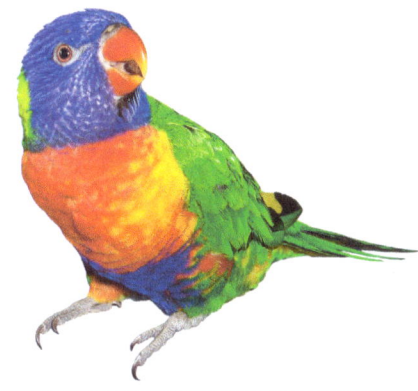

Each Laser is plugged in for different amounts of time depending on where it was in the assembly line. Just consider yourself lucky if you receive one with lots of charge already in it. This means less wait time to be able to use your Laser!

MY LASER NEEDS TO BE SHIPPED BACK FOR SERVICE. I PAID $9000 SO WILL I GET A LOANER LASER WHILE I WAIT FOR MY LASER TO BE SERVICED?

No. They do not provide a loaner Laser. Most servicing is performed quickly and the turnaround time is quite short. Even major car companies such as Toyota does not provide a loaner car despite paying $25,000 for a car. This is another reason to invest in a My Pet Laser so that you don't have to cancel any appointments while the other Laser is being serviced. Additionally, it is beneficial to Laser with two at the same time!

THE STICKER THAT COVERED A SMALL OPENING ON MY LASER CAME OFF. SHOULD I BE CONCERNED?

No. The sticker was simply covering the opening to an access port for the service department. It does not affect the function of the Laser. If the missing sticker bothers you, you may cover it with another sticker of your choice sold at many stationary stores.

I SAW THE SAME LASER BEING SOLD ON THE INTERNET FOR A BARGAIN PRICE! WHY SHOULDN'T I PURCHASE EXTRA LASERS FROM THEM?

Beware of Lasers being sold on the internet by unauthorized dealers! There are discontinued models, used, refurbished and stolen Lasers on eBay, Craig's list, Alibaba, etc. We have had several Lasers stolen and the company keeps very close records of these "hot" Lasers. They will have NO warranty! I have even seen used Lasers being sold as new - so don't be fooled! The warranty is NOT transferable even if the advertisement says it is! You don't know if the Lasers have been mistreated or how much Laser diode life is left. You won't get any service or support from these second hand Lasers not purchased directly from an official representative of the company! Support and warranty is the most important aspect of purchasing your Laser. You can't contact Amazon for a protocol on DJD, etc. Please purchase from a reputable source. BUYER BEWARE!

I HAVE A CLIENT WHO WANTS TO PURCHASE THE LASER. HOW DO I GO ABOUT THIS?

The easiest method is to refer your client to me. When your client purchases a Laser from me - you will receive a $50 Amazon eGift card as a token of thanks.

The other method is to become an Affiliate Partner and sell the Laser directly to them! You will have the opportunity to purchase the Laser at a low Affiliate Partner price. There is no inventory to carry, no minimum order quantities and I can even have the Laser drop-shipped for you. You can have your profile posted on my website to drive more new clients in your area for free! Ask me for more details on becoming an Affiliate Partner today!

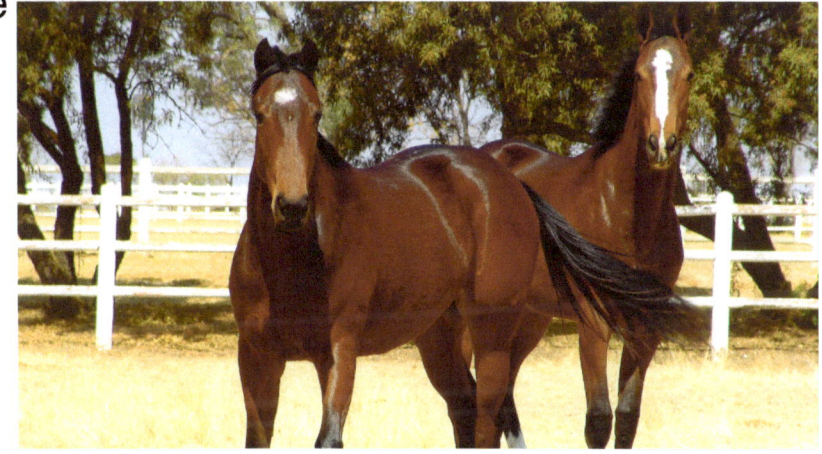

IS IT TRUE THAT I CAN RECEIVE A 10% DISCOUNT ON OVER 6000+ ACUPUNCTURE SUPPLIES?

Yes! Because you have purchased a Laser from me, I have arranged a special discount on over 6000+ acupuncture products! Ask me about this special discount on your acupuncture supplies.

SAMPLE PROTOCOLS

The following pages showcases some of the most frequently used protocols.

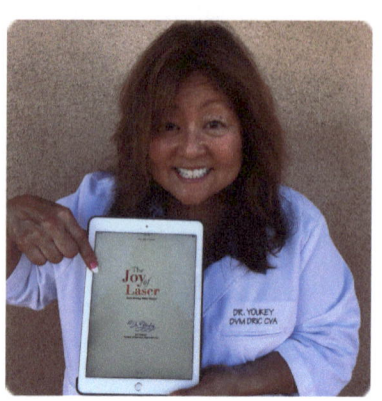

More are available on the facebook blog:

https://www.facebook.com/pg/coldlasertherapyforpetsandpeople/posts/?ref=page_internal

and in the ebook "Joy of Laser" available on Apple iBook Store:

https://books.apple.com/us/book/the-joy-of-laser/id1479515831

POST VACCINE & MICROCHIP PROTOCOL

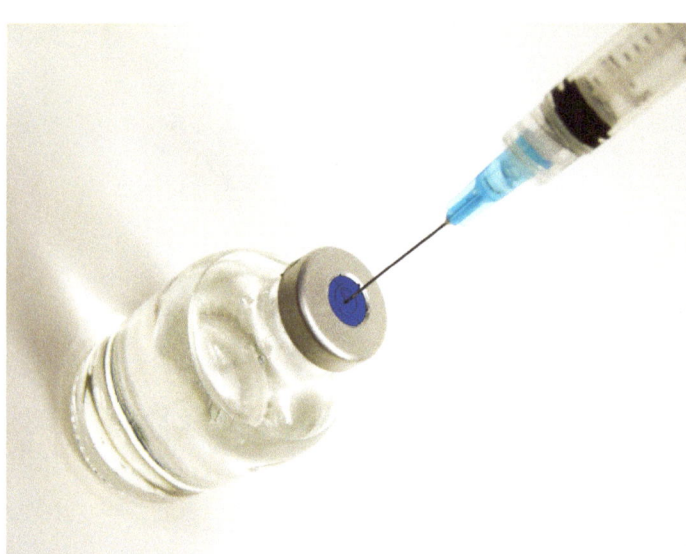

1000 Hz to stop pain immediately after the injection at the injection site. You only need to Laser a few seconds to 2 minutes. This also works on flu vaccines for humans (off-label use). You will see less vaccine reaction if you Laser after every vaccine & microchip implantation even while the patient is under anesthesia.

ARTHRITIS PROTOCOL

1000 Hz to reduce pain. Start with the unwind protocol for 2 minutes focusing in at the nerve roots along the spine associated with the arthritic area. Advance at a slow scan of 1 cm / sec to cover the arthritic area. Compress gently without eliciting pain, to push away the blood. The laser should be right against the skin or fur and you should not be able to see the red LED light as the unit is close to the body.
5 - 10 minutes depending on the severity and mass of the patient.

If there is swelling, use 1000 - 3000 Hz (variable in the TQ Solo, Pain Away or My Pet Laser) to reduce both the pain and swelling.

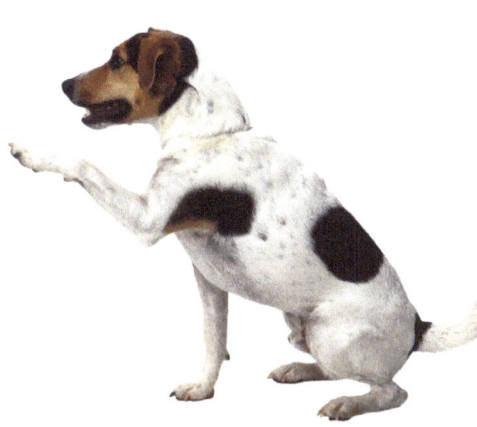

HOT SPOTS (ACRAL LICK DERMATITIS) PROTOCOL

50 Hz since we are healing. Use both the red and blue light. Start again with the unwind protocol along the associated nerve tracts along the side of the spine for 2 minutes. Then using the acupuncture probe, Laser acupuncture "circle the dragon" which is surrounding the lesion on the healthy part of the leg. You can surround the area with about 6 points and Laser for 15 seconds with the blue and red LED on. Then take the probe off and Laser over the lesion by starting first in the periphery in healthy tissue and working toward the edge and also passing over the entire wound for 2 minutes. You can Laser longer if the area is large. Do not touch the lesion, but hover as close as you to it. This is the same protocol to heal any type of wound.

OTITIS PROTOCOL

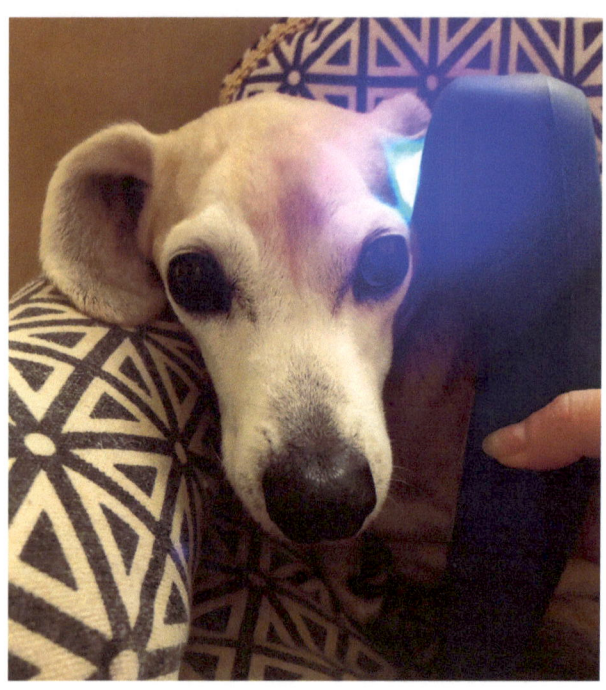

50 Hz since we are healing. Use both the red and blue light. Start again with the unwind protocol along the side of the cervical spinal column for 2 minutes. Then lift the pinnae and Laser directly into the ear canal or over the bullae from behind. Use both the red and blue LED light for 2 minutes. This patient may be ideal candidate for a rental Laser the first week.

If there is swelling and pain, use 1000 - 3000 Hz instead. Laser for 2 minutes and repeat every 4 hours.

PRE-BLOOD DRAW ANESTHETIC PROTOCOL

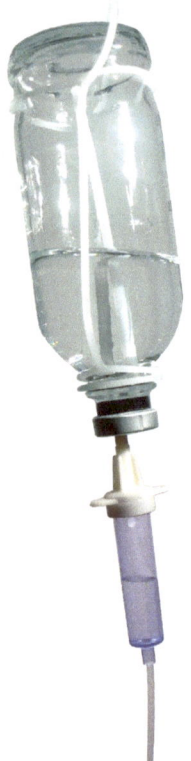

1000 Hz 1 - 2 minutes over the venipuncture site. Then once again after the blood draw to help reduce any bruising and to stop pain for another minute or less. Make sure the site has stopped bleeding before Lasering.

SNAKE BITES OR BITES OF UNKNOWN ORIGIN

A snake bite is an emergency situation and needs the expertise of the veterinarian!

Use 1000 - 3000 Hz to reduce both the pain and swelling. Please perform all the usual procedures such as fluid therapy and steroids to counter act the swelling and to maintain the patients' airways.

It would be ideal to start by Lasering the closest lymph nodes to help with lymphatic drainage. Laser over the lymph nodes for 2 minutes.

Most often the swelling is on the face. The swollen area would be too painful to compress so hover the Laser as close as you can to the affected area. Laser in a slow scan draining towards the lymph node 1 cm / sec. This means that you will be Lasering from distally to proximal. You are trying to accelerate the reduction of swelling. Repeat every 4 hours.

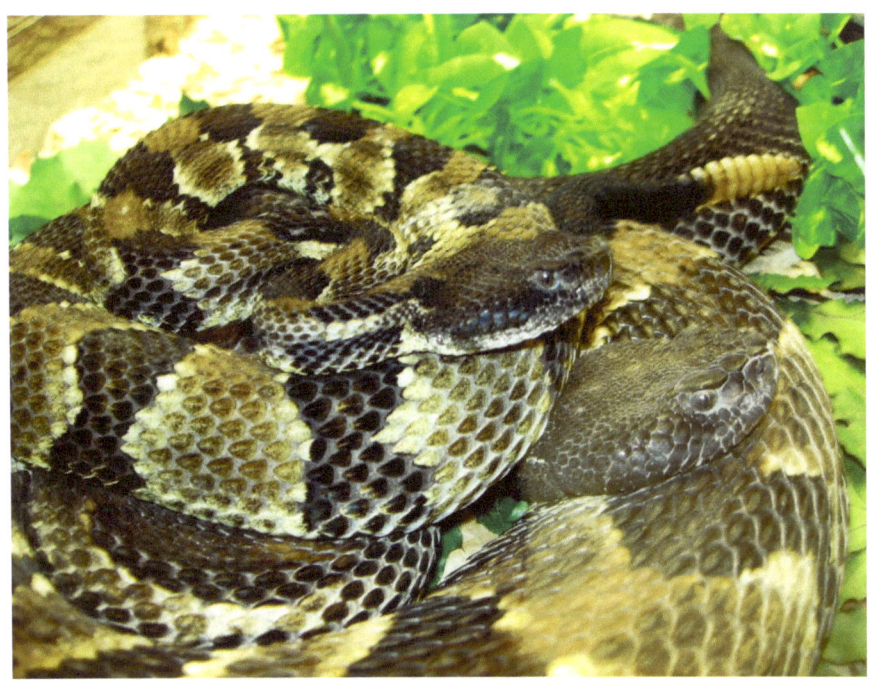

POST DE-CLAW PROTOCOL

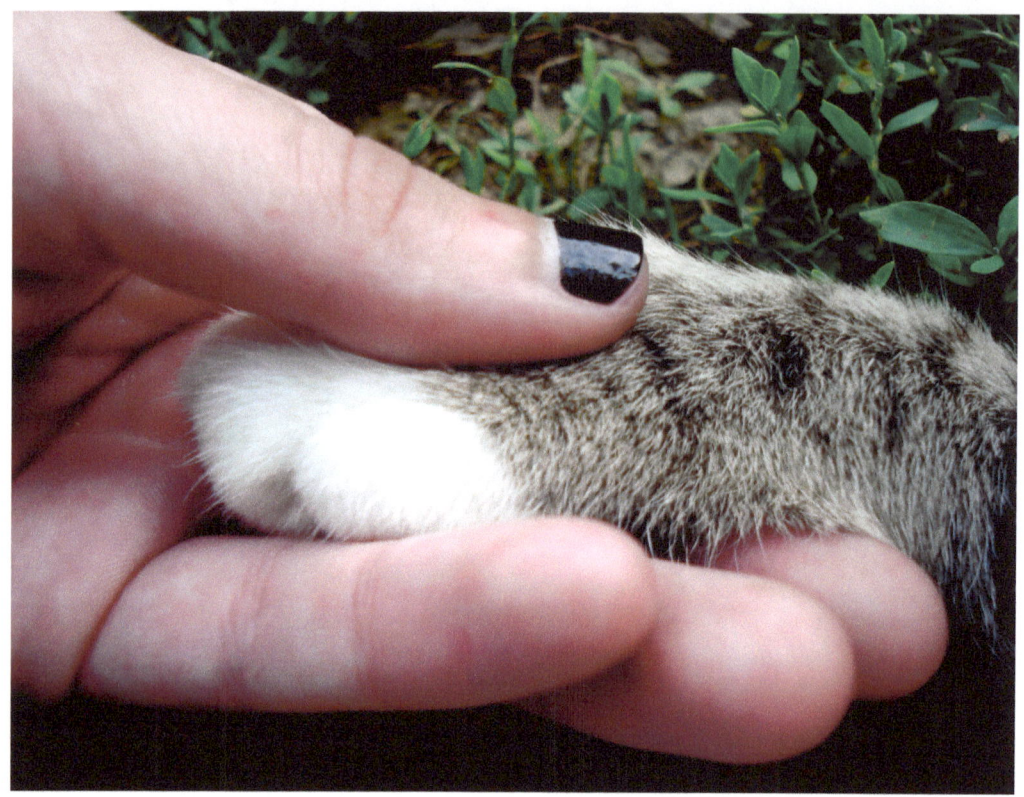

We wish this procedure were no longer performed, as this is an extremely painful procedure to recover from. Please use 1000 - 3000 Hz to help reduce their pain & swelling. Start with the unwind protocol for 2 minutes at the nerve roots along the spine associated with the declawed paws. If both the front and back legs were declawed, then be sure to Laser both the associated side of spinal column . Then a slow scan of 1 cm / sec to cover the declawed area. If the paw is small enough, you may just hold the Laser directly over the surgical area. Use both the red and blue light. Laser 5 minutes per paw while the bandage is off. Repeat every 4 hours and before the patient goes home. This is also a great time to offer the clients the rental unit so that they can continue to help reduce the pain and speed healing of their cat at home.

POST DENTAL PROTOCOL

1000 - 3000 Hz to reduce the swelling. Start with the unwind protocol along the cervical spine to stop the pain cascade to the brain for 2 minutes. If you extracted any teeth, Laser into the hole with the blue light prior to suturing for 2 minutes. Then Laser again after suturing and along the entire gum line. You can use the probes if you wish, especially if you are still using the water pik on the dental machine. Laser for 2 - 5 minutes to help accelerate the gum line healing and swelling reduction depending on the size of the mouth and how painful the procedure was on the pet.

You can cover the Laser with a Ziploc® baggie (with a desiccant placed inside) to protect it from water splashes.

For non-anesthesia teeth cleaning, run the Laser along the gum line after the polish. Use the same 1000 - 3000 Hz for 2 minutes with the red & blue light.

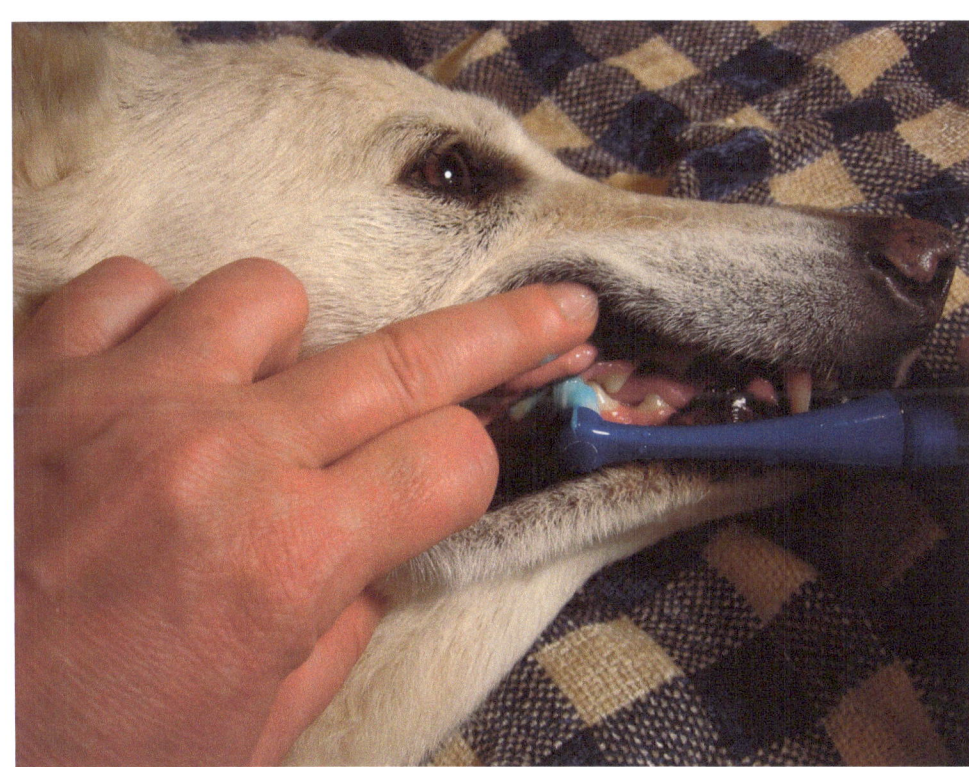

ANAL SACCULITIS PROTOCOL

50 Hz since we are healing. Use both the red and blue light. Start again with the unwind protocol along the associated nerve tracts along the side of the spine for 2 minutes. In this case, it would be the area over the sacral area. Use the trigger point probe if you need to reach into any hole. Otherwise, just use the Laser without any probes. 2 minutes treatment time with both red & blue LED on.

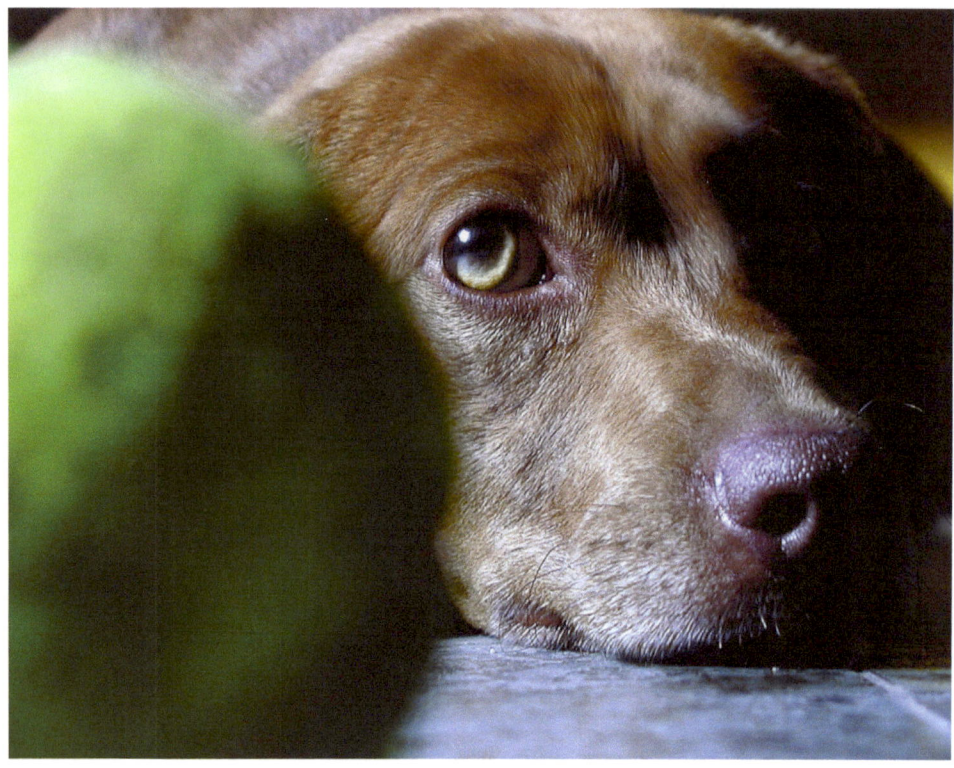

If the patient is incredibly painful and the area is swollen, I would start with the unwind protocol on 1000 -3000 Hz to stop the pain cascade to the brain. Then Instead of 50 Hz I would change to 1000 - 3000 Hz to treat for pain and swelling instead. I would still use the blue light to help kill bacteria and MRSA and Laser for 2 - 5 minutes.

If the rear area is filthy and covered in feces and pus, then place the entire Laser inside a disposable Ziploc® baggie along with a desiccant and Laser through the smoothed out plastic over the opening.

BURN PROTOCOL

Start again with the unwind protocol along the associated nerve tracts along the side of the spine for 2 minutes. But here, use 1000 Hz as we want to stop the pain cascade to the brain. Burns are terribly painful so I want to stop the pain cascade at the spinal cord, and then work on healing the burned area. If there 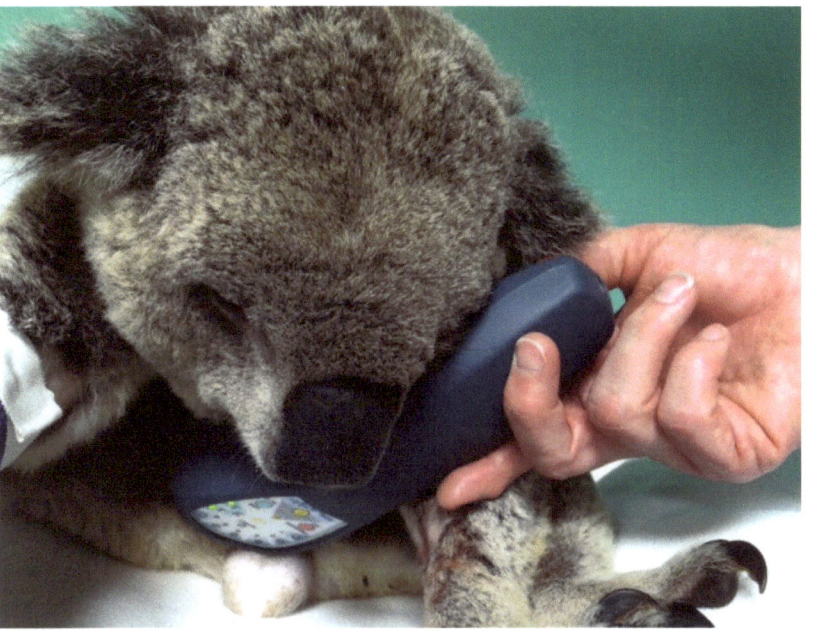 is no pain or swelling use 50 Hz to begin the healing for 2 minutes. But in the presence of pain or swelling use 1000 - 3000 Hz instead. Then make a large circle beyond the burn area to cover healthy tissue and circle around towards the middle in a slow 1 cm / sec sweep without touching the burn area (but as close as you can get). Linger longer on the healing edge. Repeat every 4 hours. These cases respond well if you have a rental unit and the owners can Laser every 4 hours, every day for the first week. Then taper off as you begin to see improvement.

Laser therapy is ideal for reptile patients suffering from thermal wounds caused by heat rocks. Reptiles have a very slow metabolism and Laser will help to accelerate their healing and reduce scar tissue formation.

These same Lasers are being utilized on the many burn victims in Australia.

CYSTITIS PROTOCOL

Use 0 - 250 Hz. The reason for this is because we want to heal but the bladder varies in depth and shape. We need to go deep as well as shallow to address the inflamed bladder wall. If the patient is in pain, then start with the unwind protocol on 1000 Hz along the spinal nerve tract associated with the bladder. Laser for two minutes to stop the pain cascade to the brain. Then switch to 0 - 250 Hz to laser directly over the bladder and also on the sides if the patient is standing to help heal the bladder. Laser for 2 minutes depending on the size of the patient.

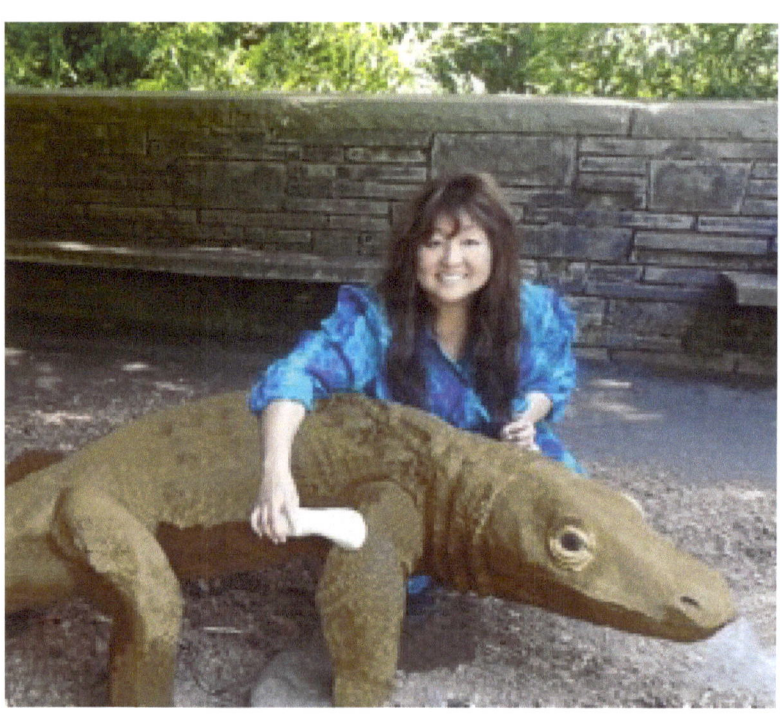

WANT MORE!?!

There's lots more protocols in my blog as well as ebooks!

Here is the link to my facebook blog with more tips:

https://www.facebook.com/pg/coldlasertherapyforpetsandpeople/posts/?ref=page_internal

The ebook "Joy of Laser" is available on Apple iBook Store:

https://books.apple.com/us/book/the-joy-of-laser/id1479515831

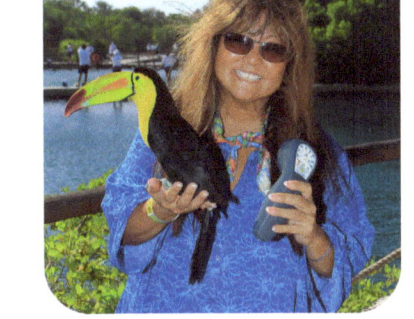

I'm here to answer all your questions, upgrade your Laser or purchase additional Lasers at the best price! Contact me at:

DRYOUKEY@MAC.COM

(303) 668-2220 text

Happy Lasering!

Dr Youkey

SURPRISE GIFT FOR YOU!

Congratulations!

Your purchase of this booklet includes a special gift!

Here is a special PROMO code that may save you money on your next Laser purchase!

PROMO CODE: GTEL

Contact me to reveal your mystery surprise!

dryoukey@mac.com

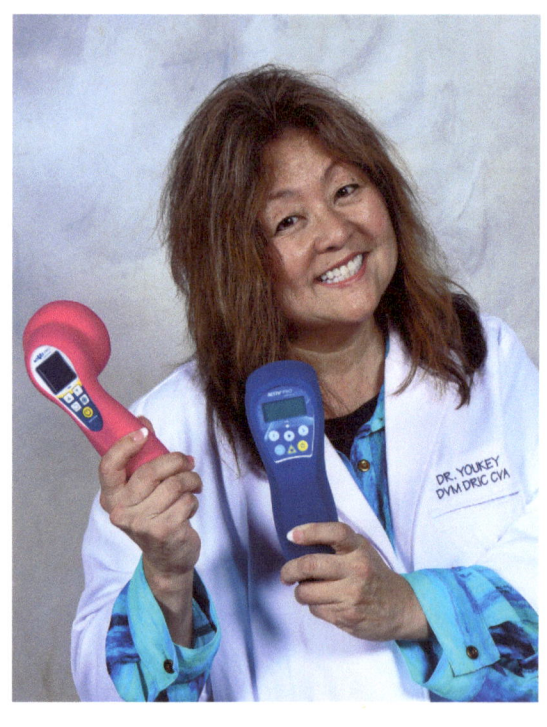

You will receive a question from this guide - that will activate the promo code above -
Oh, what fun!!!

www.ingramcontent.com/pod-product-compliance
Lightning Source LLC
Chambersburg PA
CBHW040413220526
45473CB00004B/1222